SIT-ON-TOP
KAYAKING
A BEGINNER'S GUIDE
By Tom Holtey

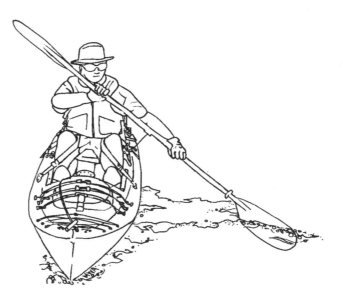

with Illustrations by
Mike Altman

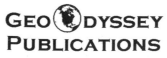

GEO ODYSSEY
PUBLICATIONS
PO BOX 25441
ROCHESTER, NY 14625

Published by GeoOdyssey Publications 1998
Printed in the United States of America

Cover photo by Doug Peebles
Page lay-out by Athena Contus

Illustrations by Mike Altman

Note: This publication is a simple guide. Please use caution in learning any new skill, especially in the outdoors where condtions are unpredictable. Be aware of appropriate and approved regulations regarding water activities in your area. Those associated with the production and writing of this book are not liable for injuries or accidents sustained by those practicing its techniques, regardless of the circumstances.

Table of Contents

ABOUT THE AUTHOR

Tom Holtey has eighteen years experience in the paddle sports industry with a foundation in canoeing and traditional sea kayaking. He has been involved in the sit-on-top field for the past nine years pioneering this new branch of the sport.

Trained and practiced in wilderness trip planning - from the White Mountains of New Hampshire and Maine to the tropical coastlines of the Hawaiian Islands - Tom, an alumni of the National Outdoor Leadership School or N.O.L.S., has lead and taught the novice adventurer under many varied conditions.

It was while teaching courses in sit-on-top kayaking at the University of Hawaii that much of this book began to take form. During this time, he managed a kayak retail store in Honolulu and worked with members of the local kayak club, Hui Wa'a Kaukahi, where many developments in the sport have been made.

Tom is currently working on more projects to promote sit-on-top kayaking and to educate those entering this growing sport.

INTRODUCTION

The Sit-on-top kayak, a new evolution of kayaking, is making this exciting outdoor pursuit available to many people who believe they lack the ability to handle a "sit-inside." This is revealed by the fact that there are three hundred thousand sit-on-top kayaks, or more, in use today.

This new generation of kayak is changing the face of the sport as we have known it. To the beginner the sit-on-top is their first exposure to kayaking. To the experienced it is something unusual. To all of us it represents a significant development in paddle sports.

Until recently, all kayakers had to learn to Eskimo-roll their boats back upright when they capsized. In sit-on-top kayaking the paddler sits on top of the kayak, instead of inside the kayak. This makes it easy to get back into and out of, therefore, tipping over is not a problem. The paddler simply rights his craft and climbs back on.

The sit-on-top, or wash deck, kayak opens this outdoor activity to people who haven't mastered the Eskimo-roll or do not care to learn it. These kayaks are also self-bailing, eliminating the need to perform a self-rescue.

Open-top kayaks are very safe and easy to paddle. This user-friendly craft provides an excellent platform for swimming, fishing, snorkeling and diving, thus expanding the use of kayaks into other fields. Sit-on-tops are also less costly than closed-deck kayaks since they do not require spray skirts, paddle floats, and a host of other accessories.

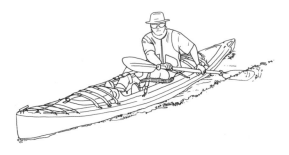

The topic of this book is to introduce the sit-on-top paddler to their craft and instruct them in the techniques and gear specific to this new generation of kayak. A glossary begins on page 85 to help you with any unfamiliar terms.

Sit-On-Top Kayaking, A Beginner's Guide is only intended to address sit-on-top issues and not kayaking as a whole. If you are seeking traditional sit-inside information you will not find it here. There are many excellent books on that subject, and I encourage you to find them. I also suggest that you attend some type of kayaking course, even if it is not for sit-on-tops. Utilize the resources of schools, dealers, clubs, symposia, outfitters and tour guides.

Any information on kayaking is valuable to both types of paddler, so read, practice experiment and share in the wonderful diversity that is available to us.

Now, let's get started...

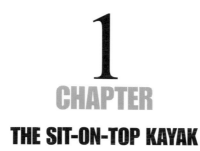

CHAPTER

THE SIT-ON-TOP KAYAK

A kayak is a one or two person watercraft that is propelled, by human power, using a double bladed paddle.

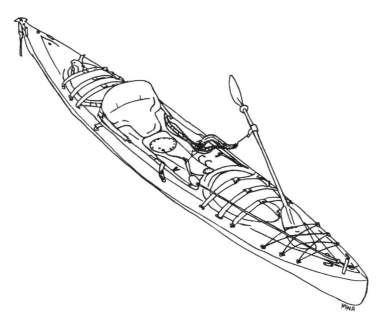

The sit-on-top kayak is similar to the sit-inside kayak. *What makes it different is the nature of the cockpit.* The cockpit is open, not enclosed by a deck and a spray skirt. A depression in the middle of the boat is the place where you sit. These kayaks are often self-bailing, using drain holes in the seat and or the feet areas. Sailors would call these *scuppers;* a nautical term defining any hole in the deck that would drain water back into the sea.

Because they are self-bailing there is no need to worry about a swamped kayak after capsizing. This makes the craft safer and easy to use. It is also easy to get into and out of.

In some conditions, like very cold weather and technical white water, a traditional kayak will be better suited and safer. In most cases, however, the sit-on-top will do the same as the sit-inside kayak.

There are differences in the accessories that are used with sit-on-top boats than with sit-inside boats. Instead of the thigh braces you use *knee straps* to grip and control the lean of the boat. The *backrest* is similar but attaches differently and often has a built in seat pad.

A *paddle leash* is more commonly used by sit-on-top paddlers than their sit-inside cousins. Many kayaks will have a *drain plug* in the bow or stern to drain bilge water.

Because of the newness of the sit-on-top kayak style, the designers of these craft have come up with some very radical designs that are changing the look of paddle sports.

This new era of kayaking is not only exciting but also expanding. New horizons are opening up to whole new groups of paddlers.

So lets go paddling
and have some fun...

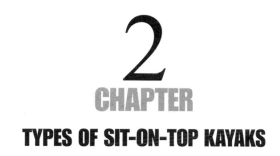

2
CHAPTER
TYPES OF SIT-ON-TOP KAYAKS

SURF SKIS: *Long slender racing kayaks*, typically eighteen-feet or more with a rudder. They are built for open ocean racing and high performance play. Surf skis are very tippy and take some practice but are the fastest kayaks on the water. If speed is what you need than this is the kayak for you.

KAYAKS: *Built for touring, camping, fishing, play, diving, surfing, snorkeling, and many more activities.* This is the most diverse category and the main topic of this book. Many styles and sizes are available. Most people will be selecting this type of craft.

WAVE SKIS: *A cross between surfboards and kayaks.* They are small flat bottom boats, six to nine feet long, with skegs or fins. This hybrid is built for riding waves, like a surfboard, but paddled like a kayak. They hydroplane down steep wave faces for an exhilarating ride, not unlike water skiing or sledding. If you are looking for excitement then gravitate to this type of sit-on-top.

INFLATABLES: *Are air filled* and can be deflated to store in a duffel bag. They are very transport-

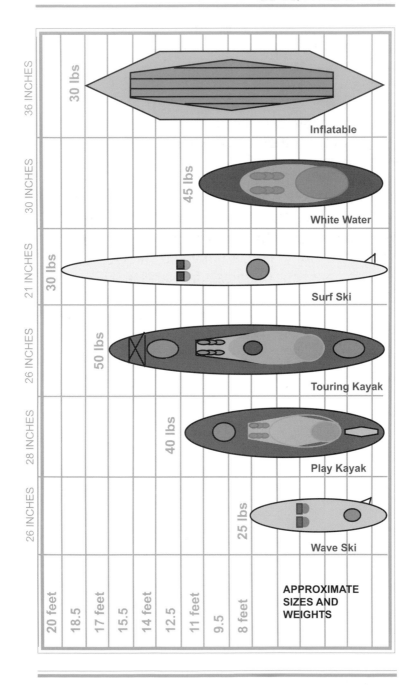

36 INCHES — 30 lbs — Inflatable

30 INCHES — 45 lbs — White Water

21 INCHES — 30 lbs — Surf Ski

26 INCHES — 50 lbs — Touring Kayak

28 INCHES — 40 lbs — Play Kayak

26 INCHES — 25 lbs — Wave Ski

20 feet | 18.5 | 17 feet | 15.5 | 14 feet | 12.5 | 11 feet | 9.5 | 8 feet

APPROXIMATE
SIZES AND
WEIGHTS

able, lightweight and stable and, in general, are used by travelers who do a lot of flying to their kayaking destinations. Inflatables have multiple chambers for safety. They can be harder to handle in windy conditions. Most take five to ten minutes to inflate with a foot or hand pump. Use these kayaks for their convenient storage and transportation.

WHITE WATER KAYAKS: *Used on rapid rivers and ocean surf.* They allow for a non-rolling paddler to venture into the river environment. Take a white water course first, so that you can read the water, choose your route carefully and know when to portage.

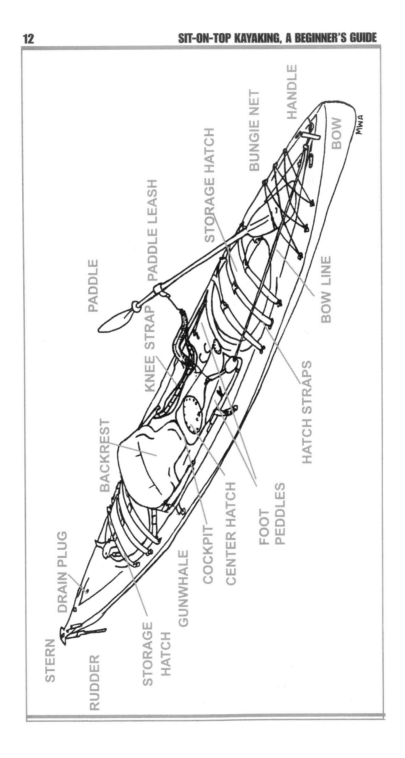

3
CHAPTER
KAYAK PARTS AND EQUIPMENT

Your kayak may be outfitted with some preinstalled features:

Handles on the bow and stern enable two people to carry the boat. They are also useful for attaching bowlines, towlines and anchor lines. A **drain plug** lets bilge water out of the kayak when you turn the boat over while on the beach.

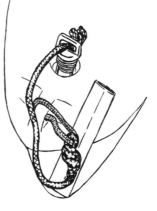

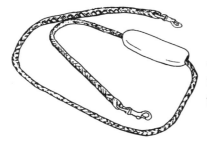

A **bowline** is a handy multipurpose rope for docking, mooring, towing and attaching the paddle leash.

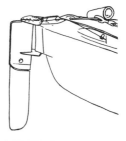

A **rudder** is a device that will help the paddler steer. It con-sists of a pivoting blade mounted on the stern at the waterline. It is connected to foot pedals in the cockpit by cables. This allows the paddler to control the angle of the rudder to turn the boat with their feet.

Your kayak may also have **storage hatches.** Hatches are openings to allow storage below deck. They may utilize lids that strap down or screw in to secure them. Some hatches are made of rubber and seal like a Tupperware. Other lids close with toggles and tabs.

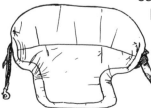

Some kayaks will have **deck lines or bungie cords** secured to the top of the kayak for gear storage or hand holds. Most kayaks will also come with accessory attachment points called **strap eyes.** These can be used for knee straps, backrests and all kinds of stuff. Sometimes there are **straps** on the deck to secure gear. Most backrests will utilize one of these straps behind the seat to attach the backrest. Many of these fea-

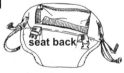

seat back

tures can be customized to fit your needs.

The **backrest** is a luxury device to add comfort to the cockpit. A well adjusted backrest can also make the kayak fit better and allow for more control, kind of like a knee strap for your behind. Most backrests attach to the sides, and behind the cockpit. Taller backrests will give more support. Shorter backrests will allow the paddler more mobility in rough water.

Knee straps are the devices that allow the paddler to get a grip on their kayak. They provide the paddler with control in surfing and rough water conditions. They are mounted on each side of the cockpit. The paddler puts the straps over their bent knees. To grip the kayak you pull your knees together. Some adjustment of the straps will be necessary. Make the knee straps tight enough so the knees do not touch, but loose enough so the legs are not spread wide. To release your self from the knee straps straighten your legs and they will fall off.

The **life vest** or **P.F.D.** (Personal Floatation Device) is the most important piece of gear. It

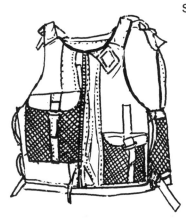

should fit comfortably but snug. Try on many different P.F.D.s before choosing one as your own. To make sure it will fit and be comfortable do these trials: Sit with the life vest on to make sure the vest will not ride up

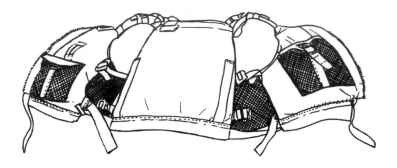

around your neck. Look for a vest with a short waistline. Swing your arms around windmill style to check for full freedom of motion. Look for a vest with large armholes. Then try the vest in the water. It should float you comfortably with out ridding up, slipping off, or rolling you face down. Use the adjustment straps to make a snug fit.

The **paddle leash** is a cord that keeps the boat and paddle together. Some look like a telephone coil. These will be very convenient, because they stay out of the way. Others are made of webbing strap; this type is very durable. Some leashes are made out of elastic. These can be fine, but beware of it snapping back at you if it is pulled tight. The leash is very helpful to beginners while they are practicing getting in and out of the kayak. The leash is also good for keeping the kayak close to you after a capsize. I recommend their use at all experience levels.

The *paddle* makes the kayak move. It consists of a shaft with a paddle blade at each end. They come in a variety of sizes, shapes and styles. *Longer paddles* are for large people and wide kayaks. *Shorter paddles* are for small people and narrow kayaks.

Blade shapes will determine the paddle's performance:

Shorter, wider, symmetrical blades are for paddlers who use a high stroke angle, with the shaft held almost vertically. This type of paddle is good for power and rough water play.

A longer asymmetrical blade is for a lower stroke angle, with the shaft held almost horizontal. This type of paddle is good for long distance and a relaxed style.

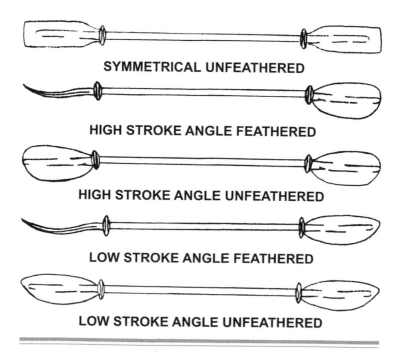

SYMMETRICAL UNFEATHERED

HIGH STROKE ANGLE FEATHERED

HIGH STROKE ANGLE UNFEATHERED

LOW STROKE ANGLE FEATHERED

LOW STROKE ANGLE UNFEATHERED

KAYAK GEAR CHECK LIST

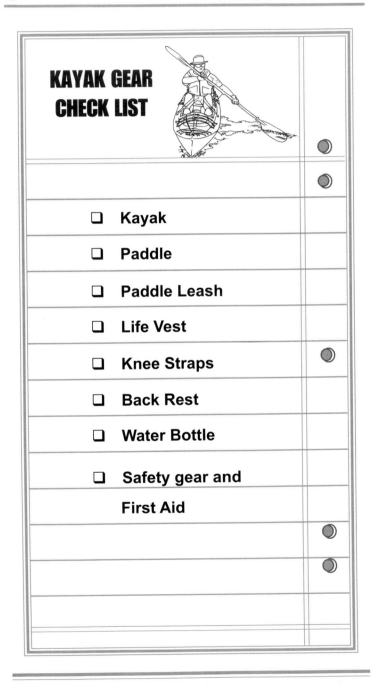

- ❑ **Kayak**
- ❑ **Paddle**
- ❑ **Paddle Leash**
- ❑ **Life Vest**
- ❑ **Knee Straps**
- ❑ **Back Rest**
- ❑ **Water Bottle**
- ❑ **Safety gear and First Aid**

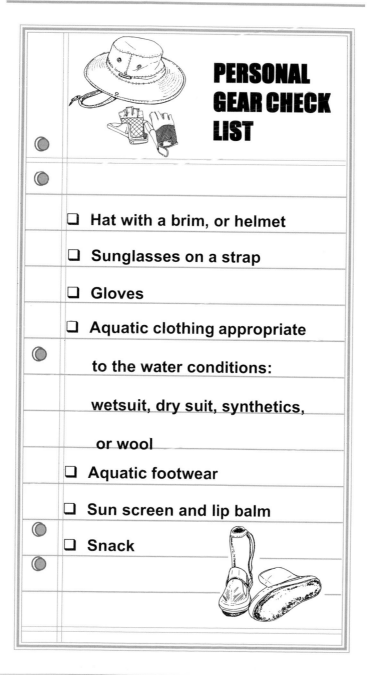

PERSONAL GEAR CHECK LIST

❑ Hat with a brim, or helmet

❑ Sunglasses on a strap

❑ Gloves

❑ Aquatic clothing appropriate

to the water conditions:

wetsuit, dry suit, synthetics,

or wool

❑ Aquatic footwear

❑ Sun screen and lip balm

❑ Snack

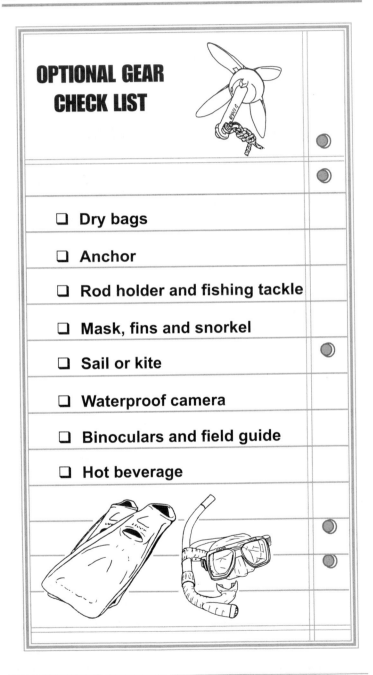

OPTIONAL GEAR CHECK LIST

- ❑ Dry bags
- ❑ Anchor
- ❑ Rod holder and fishing tackle
- ❑ Mask, fins and snorkel
- ❑ Sail or kite
- ❑ Waterproof camera
- ❑ Binoculars and field guide
- ❑ Hot beverage

CHAPTER

GETTING STARTED ON THE WATER

Before you launch your kayak check your boat and gear. Cork the drain plug, secure the hatches, make sure the accessories are properly attached, and look for any damage or defects that could cause a problem. Put on your P.F.D. Make sure that you have the appropriate personal and safety gear. *Now it is time to launch:*

GETTING IN YOUR KAYAK

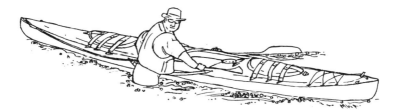

Step #1

Pull your kayak into the water, about knee to waist deep, and place your paddle clear of the cockpit. Hold your boat with both hands, one on each side of the cockpit.

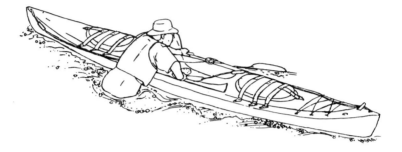

Step #2

Lift yourself up with your hands.

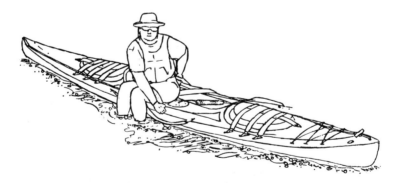

Step #3

Sit on the seat sidesaddle...

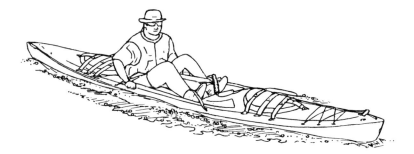

Step #4

...then place your feet into the footwells.

Pick up your paddle and take a few strokes from the shore. In more difficult conditions it may be necessary to swim the kayak out beyond the shorebreak, or you might need a push from behind by one or more people.

FALLING OFF AND GETTING BACK ON

When you fall off the kayak in deep water getting back in is easy. Just follow these steps:

1. Make sure the kayak is right side up. If not, reach under the kayak and pull the far side of the cockpit to you, and push up on the close side. This will roll the boat over right side up. Pulling on a knee strap or backrest can help. (In windy conditions you may have to roll your kayak up on the up-wind side)

Deep water entry step #1

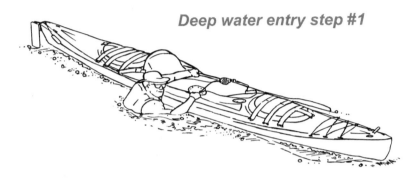

Reach for the far side of the cockpit with one hand and the close side of the cockpit with the other hand, pulling yourself across the seat area.

Deep water entry step #2

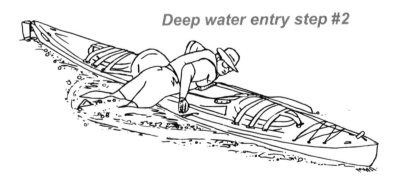

2. Flutter kicking can help propel you out of the water.

3. When your belly is on the kayak and your hips are past the gunwale, turn over so your butt slides into the seat. You should be sitting sidesaddle at this point.

Deep water entry step #3

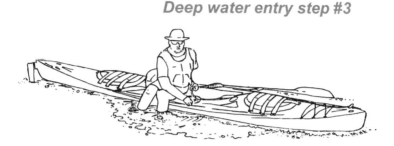

4. Lift your feet into the footwells and grab your paddle.

Deep water entry step #4

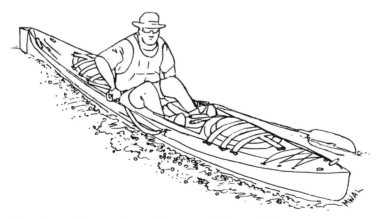

Practice these steps thoroughly and do not venture far until you have mastered them. Take your time learning to get back in your boat from deep water. It is the most important thing to learn to do.

PADDLE STROKES

GOING FORWARD

The forward stroke is done by placing the blade of
the paddle verticaly in the water near your feet.
Then...
           PUSH on the shaft
           with the upper arm, and

        PULL SLIGHTLY with the lower arm,
using back muscles for power and endurance.

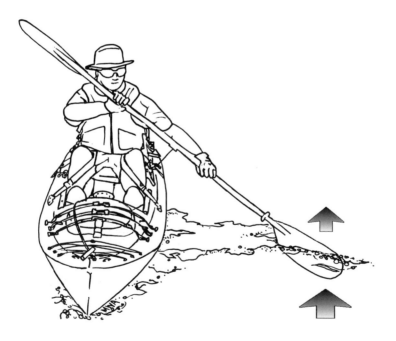

Forward stroke

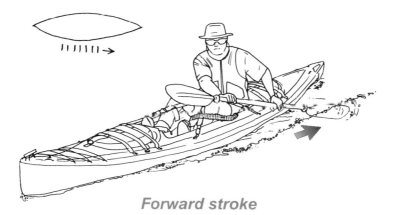

Forward stroke

Use your stomach muscles by
TURNING AT THE WAIST.
This will also enhance your stamina.

Repeat this stroke alternately
on the right and left sides,
*GIVING EQUAL FORCE
TO EACH SUCCESSIVE STROKE.*

The kayak will glide along in a straight line.

HOW TO STOP AND REVERSE

TO STOP use the forward stroke in reverse,
using the backside of the blade.
TO GO IN REVERSE keep paddling
backwards as necessary.
You can even use the paddle as a rudder off the
bow to fine-tune your direction.

USING A FEATHERED PADDLE

The beginning paddler will often be mysti-
fied by the feathered paddle. Most paddles can be
feathered or unfeathered by adjusting a center
connector in the shaft.

The unfeathered paddle has blades that
are parallel. Use of this type of paddle is very
intuitive and requires no special technique.

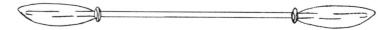

The feathered paddle, however, has
blades that are as much as forty-five to ninety
degrees offset. Grip it tight with the right hand and
loose with the left hand (Left handed people can
do the reverse.)

The right wrist controls the angle of the

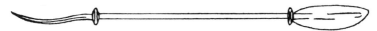

blade. Hold your paddle out in front of you like the
handle bar of a motorcycle. Turn the "accelerator"
on by twisting your right wrist. Let the shaft turn
freely in the left hand.

**Imagine glue in your right hand and
grease in your left hand.** The shaft and blades
will rotate. You are now controlling the angle of the
blade.

Incorporate this into your technique. Take a
stroke with the right blade, rotate the shaft to
realign the left blade and take another stroke on
the left, then rotate the shaft back and take a

stroke on the right side. Keep repeating this and you are paddling feathered.

The reason for the feathered paddle is wind resistance. The returning blade cuts through the air as the other blade pushes on the water. In a strong head wind this can save a lot of energy.

TURNING AND STEERING

TO MAKE SMALL COURSE CORRECTIONS

While going forward, you can use your paddle like a rudder by dragging it slightly just behind you.

The blade should be in a vertical position, without using too much backward pressure or forward momentum will be lost.

The rudder stroke can also be used in reverse at the bow while going backwards.

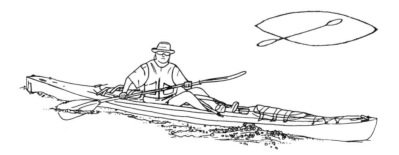

Rudder stroke

THE SWEEP STROKE WILL ALLOW YOU TO MAKE SHARP TURNS.

Place the paddle near your feet,
like the forward stroke,
but sweep the water in a wide arc,
away from the side and toward the stern.
This will make the boat turn to the opposite side.

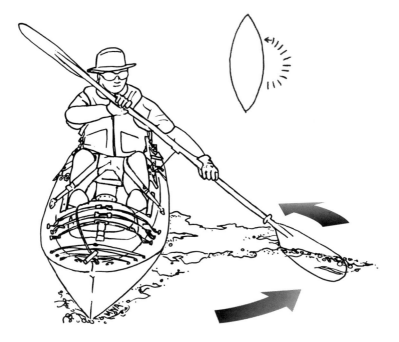

SWEEP STROKE

You can also use this stroke in reverse to cause the kayak to turn in reverse.

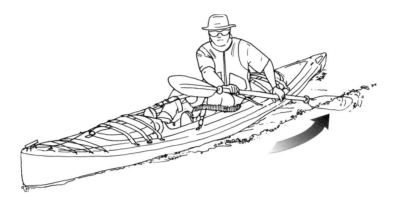

Sweep stroke

TO PIVOT THE KAYAK...

USE A FORWARD SWEEP ON ONE SIDE AND A REVERSE SWEEP ON THE OTHER SIDE.

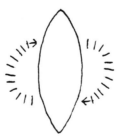

This will make the boat spin,
with you in the center.

GOING SIDEWAYS

TO MAKE YOUR KAYAK GO SIDEWAYS, USE THE DRAW STROKE.

This stroke can be used to pull up along side a dock or other kayaker.

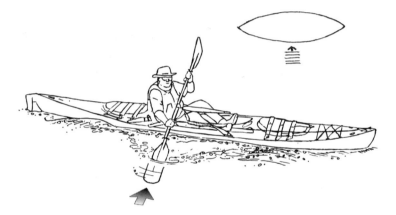

Draw stroke

PLACE YOUR PADDLE OUT TO ONE SIDE AS FAR AS YOU CAN COMFORTABLY REACH.

PULL THE BLADE TOWARD YOU, LIKE RAKING LEAVES.

SLICE THE BLADE OUT OF THE WATER...

before it comes too close to the boat,
by lowering the upper hand until the shaft
is parallel to the water's surface.

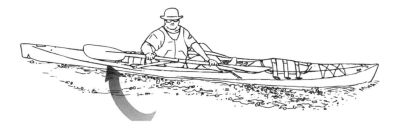

Draw stroke

IF YOU DO NOT TAKE THE BLADE OUT OF THE WATER IT WILL CONTINUE MOVING UNDER THE HULL AND PULL YOU IN AFTER IT.

MAINTAINING STABILITY

Bracing can keep you from tipping over.

To brace, slap the blade on the water
with a quick shallow whack.
You can push down to stay up,
just like you can push back to go forward.

You can not lean on the paddle as it will
sink down into the water. Keep the blade shallow.
Be ready to brace instantly on the opposite side if
you use this stroke too vigorously, or if the water is
really rough.
      This is an important stroke to practice. Rock
your kayak from side to side, and slap the water
on each side, gripping tightly on your knee straps
with your legs. Do this for a few minutes until it has
become an automatic response. If you do not
capsize while doing this exercise, you are not
trying hard enough.

PROPER LEAN OF THE BOAT AT THE HIPS IS VERY IMPORTANT.

      Your hips should lean and tilt with the boat
like a hula dancer's hips.The upper body and head
should always be directly over the centerline.
      If you let your upper body swing like a
metronome, you will tip over.
      If you let your waist be junction of the rock-
ing lower body and the stable upper body then you
will not tip over (as much).

TRY THIS EXERCISE:

Wiggle your hips like hula dancing keeping the body strait up and down.

Make the boat rock side to side using only the lower body so that waves go out in rows on each side of your boat.

Now you are "hip snapping."

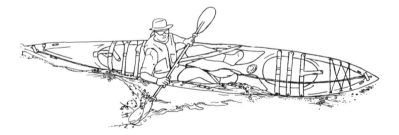

Brace stroke

PROPER LEAN OF THE BOAT
WITH THE HIPS IS VERY IMPORTANT.

LANDING AND LAUNCHING ON THE SHORE

To land, paddle to the shore. The water at the shoreline can be surprisingly rough, and can cause an ungraceful capsize. For that reason, before you get to the beach, hop off the kayak in water about waist deep. Then quickly pull it by the bow, up the beach to the high water mark before any waves push it around.

Try to stay on the ocean side of the boat in the shore break so that the kayak will not strike you in the shins when it is pushed by the waves.

Sometimes in rough conditions it is necessary to have some people help hold the kayak while in the surf zone.

When paddling in a group, have the most experienced person land first. Then he or she can help the others land one at a time. Reverse this procedure for launching. In calm water you will not need to take these precautions.

See "*GETTING IN YOUR KAYAK*" for details of launching on the shore.

LANDING AND LAUNCHING ON A DOCK

To launch from a dock, place the paddle on the dock surface and just behind the seat of your kayak so it makes a bridge, from dock to deck.

Then sit on the dock with your feet in the cockpit of your kayak. Place your hands on the paddle, behind you, with one over the kayak and the other over the dock.

Put your weight on the paddle shaft while

you shift your butt from the dock to the seat of
your boat. Reposition your paddle in front of you
and push away gently, then begin paddling.

To land on a dock, pull up to the dock
sideways. Place your paddle behind you so that it
is resting on the back deck and the dock surface,
making a bridge.

Put one hand on the paddle behind you
over the kayak and the other hand on the paddle
over the dock surface. Your weight should be on
your paddle.

Lift your butt off the seat and onto the dock.
Then lift your feet out of the cockpit an on to the
dock. Tie the kayak promptly so it will not drift
away.

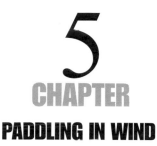

5

CHAPTER

PADDLING IN WIND

Wind is the worst enemy of the kayaker. On days with strong winds...

➤ paddle only in protected waters.
➤ always plan your trips with the prevailing wind directions in mind.

If you plan a trip where you start and end in the same place...

➤ paddle against the wind first, then return with the wind at your back.

This way you will have the wind helping you when you are the most tired.

If planning a trip with a different put in and take out, then plan to go with the wind at your back.

Use caution while paddling on a coast with an offshore wind. Do not paddle so far offshore that paddling back to shore will be too difficult. Use caution also while paddling with an onshore wind. Paddle far enough offshore so that you will not be pushed ashore. This can be very important on a rocky coast with breaking waves.

Always be aware of the wind direction and strength. Anticipate how the kayak will be pushed by the wind and adjust your course and plans appropriately.

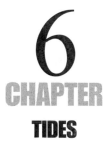

6

CHAPTER

TIDES

Tides are the movements of the ocean waters due to the gravitational forces of the moon.

The water at the ocean shoreline will rise and fall two times a day. This can cause strong currents where ocean waters ebb and flow...

- ➤ through narrow channels,
- ➤ in and out of bays and inlets,
- ➤ around points of land.

These currents are best avoided.

Use a tide chart and pilots book to determine the best time of day to paddle. The knowledge of local, experienced paddlers will be invaluable.

If you do find yourself paddling in a tidal flow (or river) you may need to ferry across the current by pointing your kayak upstream and slightly toward your destination.

This will allow you to paddle against the current while at the same time maintain your course.

When your kayak is beached on shore, make sure that the tide will not come up and float your boat away on the current. It is recommended that you pull your kayak up past the high water mark and tie it off.

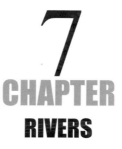

CHAPTER
RIVERS

Paddling on flat-water rivers is not particularly difficult. White water rivers, however, are very dangerous. Training from certified instructors is mandatory. It is not recommended for any one to paddle in white water without this training.

Flat-water rivers, without fast currents, obstacles, and waterfalls, do not require extensive training. You should be aware of:

> ➢ the current
> ➢ it's rate of flow
> ➢ where it is taking you.

Know what lies ahead. Dams, waterfalls, rapids and steep banks with no take out, are the dangers to look for. Some flat-water rivers flow slow enough to paddle up or down stream. Other rivers will allow only down stream paddling. Some rivers have both slow and fast moving sections.

The water level of a river can change. When landing always pull your kayak up past the high water mark and/or tie it off to something.

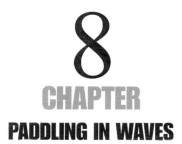

8

CHAPTER

PADDLING IN WAVES

Waves can be a formidable foe, but in the right conditions can also provide excellent practice.

When paddling out through waves, keep your kayak pointed right at them. Your kayak is more stable from bow to stern than it is from side to side.

The larger the wave coming at you the harder you must paddle to climb the face of the wave. If you are not paddling fast enough, the wave will push you back to shore, and possibly capsize you.

When returning back through the waves, keep your kayak pointed to shore. The waves will help you back to shore. Your kayak will want to go sideways and roll like a log to the beach. To prevent this, you must steer your kayak using your paddle like a rudder. If you steer too much on one side, your boat will go sideways. It is necessary to steer a little bit on one side and then a little bit on the other side, constantly counter steering until the ride is over.

Avoid high surf. Small to medium waves can be quite fun, but they can also throw you off your kayak and sweep it away from you. Once the kayak is sideways there is little you can do to correct it. You can prevent your boat from rolling over by bracing your paddle on the wave face while leaning toward the wave. Hold on tight to the knee straps with your legs, and lean the hull of your kayak so that the bottom will act as a buffer, striking any obstacles in the surf zone.

9
CHAPTER
DRIVING YOUR KAYAK HOME

Putting your kayak on top of your car to transport it is often a subject that is overlooked. You can put any size kayak on any size car.

Get a good roof rack system that works well with your car. Choose foam soft racks or metal hard racks.

The kayak should be tied to the roof rack with straps, and to the front and back bumpers of your car, or in some cases to the roof of the car through the doors.

To test your tie downs, shake the kayak vigorously, if the car shakes with it and they both

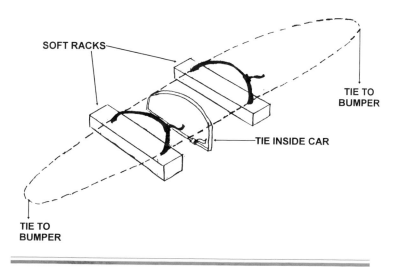

SOFT RACKS

TIE TO BUMPER

TIE INSIDE CAR

TIE TO BUMPER

move as one then the tie down is good. If the boat is loose then you must retighten the tie downs. Drive with caution and be careful of low over-hangs.

Some people will have trouble lifting the kayak up onto the roof. You can purchase accessories from roof rack manufactures that can assist you, like rollers and extensions.

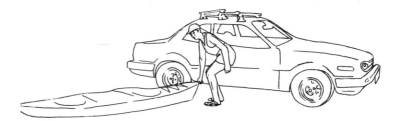

LIFT BOW BY HANDLE... LEAN IT ON THE RACK...

You can also lift one end of the kayak up onto the rack, one half the weight of the boat, and then from the other end of the kayak, lift and position the boat on the rack. You can use this procedure in reverse to take the kayak down.

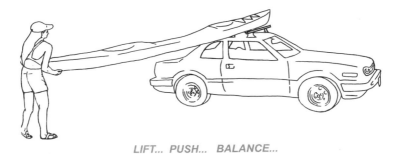

LIFT... PUSH... BALANCE...

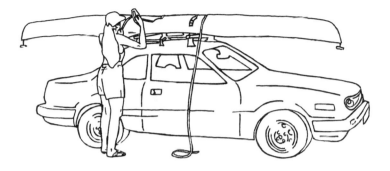

FLIP THE KAYAK OVER SO THAT THE COCKPIT RESTS ON THE RACK AND RESISTS SLIDING FORWARD OR BACKWARD.

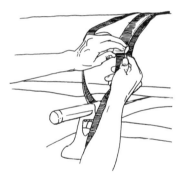

TIE SECURELY

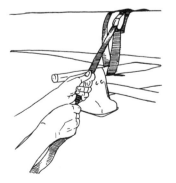

10
CHAPTER

NOW THAT YOU ARE KAYAKING

Now that you are familiar with the basics of kayaking you can expand into the many branches of the sport. You can use kayaks for camping, racing, surfing, diving, snorkeling, fishing, exercise, day trips, commuting, and communing with nature. The only limits are your imagination.

FISHING

Fishing and hunting were the original uses of kayaks by Eskimos. Kayak means "hunter's boat" in the Eskimo language.

To fish from your kayak you will need your basic fishing gear. Keep it simple in the beginning. Make sure you store the tackle in the hatch or some other secure place so it won't go overboard.

Trolling can be done by trailing a fishing lure behind your kayak. You can use a rod or a hand line. If you use a rod you will need a rod holder installed on the deck. It should be placed ahead of the paddler near the feet but some folks prefer installing their rod holders behind the seat.

Angle the rod holder out to one side so that the rod is reaching out overboard, or overhead.

Deploy your line with a selected lure or bait. Keep your speed up so the lure won't snag the bottom. A floating lure is very handy for this reason.

It is a good idea to tie the rod to the kayak so it can't sink if you tip over. Use a paddle leash or string long enough for this so you can have freedom of motion while you are playing the fish.

Bottom fishing and casting are also popular ways to fish from your kayak. Some people use an anchor to stay in one place while others prefer to drift.

When you catch your fish you may need to straddle your kayak for extra stability. Once you have landed your catch put it and any other loose tackle away in a safe place so it will not go overboard.

UNDERWATER ADVENTURES

Diving and snorkeling from a kayak is convenient and safe. You won't have to swim long distances to your dive site and you will have a safety platform to rest on if you need it.

Use an anchor or a long towrope to secure your kayak. A good anchor line will be very long, more than double or triple the depth of the water you wish to moor in. If you wish to use a towrope, 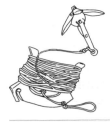 it should be something you hold in you hand, or have a "quick release," to prevent entanglement.

Keep your dive gear in a mesh deck bag or tie it to the deck so it won't fall over board. You can also put you gear in the hatches of your boat.

When opening hatches, get your stuff out and promptly close the lid when you are done. Do not open hatches in rough water.

A bilge pump is handy to have if water gets into your hull while the boat is open. A bilge pump is an important safety device for those who need to do a lot of loading and unloading of heavy objects while in deep water.

Scuba divers will want to assemble their scuba unit on the beach before launching. Put on your wet suit, leaving the top open and the arms tied around your waist. The scuba unit should be securely strapped into a dive tankwell on the kayak or put into a hatch.

Once you are at your dive site, deploy your anchor first. Put the scuba unit over board, by pulling it up to your hip and sliding it down one leg, like a boat ramp. Tie it promptly to the kayak. Then pull on your wet suit and don the rest of your gear.

A dive flag is necessary to warn other boaters of your presence. Put up your dive flag before entering the water.

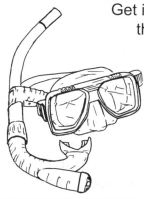

Get into your scuba unit while in the water. Then make your descent by following the anchor line. Make sure your anchor is secure. The anchor makes a good underwater landmark. Start your navigation from here.

When it is time to ascend, start at your

anchor and make sure it will be easy to retrieve. For deep, long, or multiple dives place a mark on your line at fifteen feet for a safety stop.

When you surface, swim to the kayak and get out of the scuba unit while in the water. Tie the tank to the kayak so that it will not drift away. Knee straps can do double duty as gear tethers.

Get back on and remove the rest of your dive gear and stow it securely. With your legs overboard for stabil- ity, pull the scuba unit up one leg and then slide it into its storage place. Use care not to damage the hatch gaskets. Secure equipment with the gear straps or hatch lid.

The last thing to do is to pull up the anchor. If the anchor becomes stuck on something down there, then it may be necessary to paddle into the wind a little bit to tug the anchor in the other direc- tion to dislodge it.

SURFING

Kayak surfing is an excellent pursuit for those wanting a thrill. The surf zone is also a challenge to those launching and landing on beaches that are exposed to open ocean conditions. It is good for non-surfers to practice in the surf zone for rough water experience.

TO SURF YOUR KAYAK:

➤Sowly paddle shoreward with the waves coming from behind.

➤Keep your attention out to sea so you can watch for waves and not be taken by surprise.

➤Select a wave and get your kayak moving by taking short shallow strokes at a fast rate. This will increase acceleration and make it easy to catch the wave.

➤Once on the wave you may need to lean back to prevent your kayak from taking a nosedive.

➤By leaning back you will slow down.

➤By leaning forward you will speed up.

Your kayak will want to turn sideways to the wave on its own accord. To overcome this natural action you must control its direction. When using

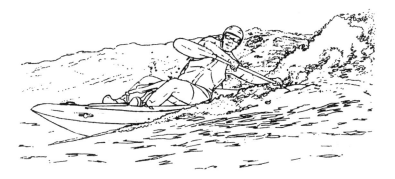

small surfing kayaks lean to the side that you want to turn to. Grip your knee straps tightly with your legs to keep on top of the kayak and to fine tune your lean. Place your paddle flat on the water just

behind you on the side you want to turn toward.
The paddle will start to surf like a small surfboard.

By bracing like this you can put weight on
the paddle and make your kayak lean more. The
kayak will continue to turn to that direction until
you counter steer and lean on the other side.

To keep straight on your chosen course,
you must steer on one side and then the other
side. You must constantly counter steer to keep
the boat on your intended path. Once your ride is
over, turn around and find a route out to the take
off zone. Keep out of the rough water and the path
of other surfers.

If you start to go sideways on the wave,
or otherwise become broached, then brace on
the wave face and lean into it. Riding the wave
sideways while on top is better than letting the
wave roll you and your kayak over like a log. Hold
on tight with your knee straps. Use your hips to
angle the hull so that the kayak hydroplanes down
the wave face on its edge. Allow the bottom of the
boat to lead, it will protect your body from colli-
sions. The hull will take the impact and you won't.

Longer touring kayaks are harder to control,
but easy to catch the wave. The steering is different. Use your paddle like a rudder. You will also
need to counter steer continuously like the small
surf boats. This takes some strength and skill. If
your touring kayak has a rudder this will help
control the boat on the wave face considerably,
however rudders can be damaged in strong waves
while broaching.

When you capsize in the surf zone it is
best to grip tightly on the knee straps with your

legs, tuck your head down to your knees and place the paddle along one side of the boat, maintaining your regular grip.

Sometimes the kayak will right itself by the natural rolling motion of the wave. By holding this position you will be ready to brace when you turn upright and come to the surface. At the very least this position will prevent the kayak from getting away from you.

If you can not hold your breath, then straighten out your legs and the knee straps will fall off leaving you free to find sweet air. Hold onto the paddle. It is attached to the paddle leash and thus to the kayak. This will prevent you from having to swim after your kayak, and will allow you to still maintain some control over it.

Surfing can be challenging and dangerous. I recommend wearing a helmet and your PFD. Scout out the break to find any hazards, like shallow reef, rip tides, or under water rocks.

Always use caution. Do not surf in conditions that are beyond your ability. The most important thing to accomplish in the surf zone is to stay on top of the kayak. Bracing and hip control is crucial.

Getting through the surf zone is something worth practicing even if you are not planing to be a surf kayaker. Try getting broached on purpose. Paddling out through waves and trying to maintain position in the surf zone is a great aerobic exercise. Riding the waves is more than just an exhilarating ride. It is also excellent practice.

CAMPING EXPEDITIONS

Camping from a kayak is one of the most rewarding of the boating experiences. You can use your kayak to venture into remote areas that few people have the opportunity to visit. The feeling of freedom and self-sufficiency is wonderful.

Plan your camping trips well. Preparation makes the trip easier and safer. Day trips need planning also, and they are excellent practice for expeditions.

Choose a route

Consult someone experienced with the territory and seasonal weather conditions. Get a guide book for the region. Make sure the distances you must travel are realistic for every one in the group. Plan spots along the way for emergency landings, rest stops, and lunch places.

Permits

Check with state and county agencies to obtain any necessary permits or regulations. Also check with owners of private property that you might want to camp on or explore.

Test load your gear

Bring regular camping gear and store it all in waterproof bags. You should test load your gear to make sure it will all fit in your kayak and the dry bags.

Load the heavy stuff in the middle of the kayak, and the lighter stuff in the ends. It is best to load the boat evenly or heavier to the rear. In some cases, with a strong head wind or while paddling into a strong current, you might want to put a little more weight toward the front.

Launching and landing

A fully loaded kayak will be heavy, so load it near the water's edge.

When you have found your campsite, make sure that your kayaks are pulled well above the high water mark and tied to a tree or rock. Tides and waves are notorious for taking unattended boats away from their owners and leaving them stranded without transportation. This can even happen on a river or lake with changing water levels. Make sure that your kayaks are secure no matter how short you plan to make your stay.

Finally, please carry out every thing that you bring into the wilderness. Try to leave no trace that you were there.

CAMPING GEAR LIST

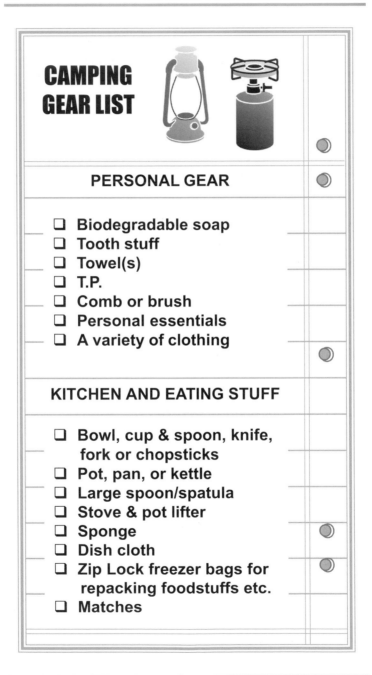

PERSONAL GEAR

- ☐ Biodegradable soap
- ☐ Tooth stuff
- ☐ Towel(s)
- ☐ T.P.
- ☐ Comb or brush
- ☐ Personal essentials
- ☐ A variety of clothing

KITCHEN AND EATING STUFF

- ☐ Bowl, cup & spoon, knife, fork or chopsticks
- ☐ Pot, pan, or kettle
- ☐ Large spoon/spatula
- ☐ Stove & pot lifter
- ☐ Sponge
- ☐ Dish cloth
- ☐ Zip Lock freezer bags for repacking foodstuffs etc.
- ☐ Matches

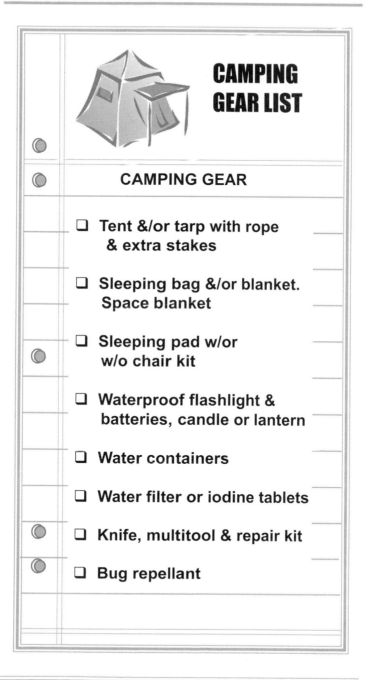

CAMPING GEAR LIST

CAMPING GEAR

- ❏ Tent &/or tarp with rope & extra stakes

- ❏ Sleeping bag &/or blanket. Space blanket

- ❏ Sleeping pad w/or w/o chair kit

- ❏ Waterproof flashlight & batteries, candle or lantern

- ❏ Water containers

- ❏ Water filter or iodine tablets

- ❏ Knife, multitool & repair kit

- ❏ Bug repellant

11

ROUTE PLANNING

Planning your route ahead of time is essential, particularly if it is unfamiliar territory.

You will need a map, tide charts, guide book, and some working knowledge of local weather conditions, tides, and currents. If on a river, research the location of rapids and portages. Where available, check the surf or river report. Have a basic plan in mind, such as a destination.

TO PLAN YOUR ROUTE:

Look at your map and find your starting point and your destination. Apply your knowledge of currents, tides and wind direction to the map.

It is best to have the winds, currents, and tides in your favor. Paddling against the current, wind, or tide can be hard to impossible.

Look for lunch and rest stops. Apply your working knowledge of wave directions to determine if the landings will be rough or not. If you are on a river identify any rapids and portages. Carefully note which side of the river the portage is on.

You may also want to identify a couple of regrouping areas for your party to gather at if you should begin to spread out or need a group meeting. This can be on the water if you can find a calm bay, protected lee, or section of slow moving water on a river.

Finally, make notes on your plan, and put them, the map, and any other pertinent information in a waterproof see through map case. This will allow you to easily refer to your plan while on the water. It would be best if everyone in the group had a map case with this information, but at least the lead and sweep kayakers should carry copies.

Safe Kayaking Check List

THIS IS A LIST OF SAFETY EQUIPMENT THAT ALL SIT-ON-TOP KAYAKERS SHOULD CARRY

- ❏ PFD or "life vest" (coast guard approved)
- ❏ Drinking water in waterproof container
- ❏ Paddle leash &/or leg leash, & life line
- ❏ Bilge pump
- ❏ Knife
- ❏ Signal devices: whistle, signal mirror, flare, smoke, dyemarker, See Rescue, air horn
- ❏ Cell phone &/or radio in waterproof bag or "CellSafe"
- ❏ Spare paddle
- ❏ Proper clothing, aquatic foot wear & hat
- ❏ Flash light (waterproof) &/or strobe light for dusk or night
- ❏ Tow rope
- ❏ Helmet for surfing, rock gardens, seacaves & whitewater rivers
- ❏ Float bags
- ❏ Repair kit: duct tape, spare parts, tools, etc.
- ❏ Sea anchor
- ❏ Sun screen
- ❏ Sting aid
- ❏ First Aid kit

Carry as many of these devices as possible &
KNOW HOW TO USE THEM.
PRACTICE
with them in a variety of weather conditions so you
can use this equipment no matter how bad it gets.
BE SAFE.
Always go with a buddy, and tell some one who cares
where you are going, what you are going to do and
when you will be back. Plan ahead and
BE PREPARED.

12

CHAPTER

SAFETY

Safety is a concern to all boaters. Common sense and proper procedures will eliminate most unfortunate situations. Educate yourself about possible hazards you may encounter while on the water. Prepare your plans and equipment. Know your limitations.

Personal Safety

Planning, preparation and maintenance are the keys to good safety protocol. Inspect your equipment regularly for defects and damage.

Leaks are the most critical thing to look for. Check the hull of your kayak for cracks. Inspect the seals of your hatches for wear. Also look for a worn or poorly fitting drainplug.

Even a broken strap eye can cause a performance problem if it prevents the use of your knee straps. Take care of this before you are on the beach while your companions are waiting. Use your safety checklist to make sure that all the necessary equipment is ready and in good shape.

Group Safety

Group organization is essential in order to minimize any confusion or miscommunications. A **float plan** is a good place to start.

The plan should consider...

> ➤where and when you will be paddling
> ➤the starting place
> ➤the ending place
> ➤the route your group will take
> ➤alternative routes or landings
> ➤how many people are going
> ➤who they are

Regular head counts are a good idea. Then, finally let a responsible person, who is not going on your trip, know of the plan.

It would help if the plan were in writing. Everyone in the group needs to know the plan as well. Have a group meeting prior to launch to make the plan clear to all members. At this time a lead kayaker and a sweep kayaker should be chosen.

The lead kayaker should be a strong paddler, with experience and a good idea of where you are going. It is his job to lead the group, mak- ing decisions on where to go and where not to go. The lead kayaker should paddle at a pace that everyone in the group can sustain and no one in the group should pass him or her.

The sweep kayaker should also be a strong experienced paddler who is inclined to paddle at a slower pace. The sweep should have a well-stocked supply of safety and signal devices. It will most likely be the sweep who will have to assist a paddler in distress. They should have experience in kayak rescue techniques. It is the responsibility of the sweep paddler not to let anyone fall behind them. The sweep should keep an eye out for the paddlers ahead of them and maintain the pace of the slowest paddler.

It is helpful if the lead and the sweep can communicate via radio or cell phone. Then those in front will know what the back is doing and the back will know what the front is doing. Of course, it is best to keep the group close together, but in some conditions that can be hard to do.

Good safety protocol not only will help prevent disaster, but will enhance your enjoyment of the sport and create group camaraderie.

13
CHAPTER

KAYAK RESCUES

The ability to perform a rescue, and a self-rescue, is very important. Help will not always be readily available.

Rescue procedures should be learned in a controlled environment and practiced under the conditions that you plan to paddle in. You will then be familiar with the techniques, should the need arise.

EXCESS BILGE WATER

The most important procedure to learn is the management of bilge water in your kayak. A little water in the kayak is not usually a problem. A lot of water is a problem. Rough water, heavy loads, old boats and inexperienced paddlers are usually the causes of excess bilge water.

Every kayak should have a means of bailing. The best bailer is a bilge pump. A sponge or a small bucket will suffice in a pinch.

Should your kayak feel a little tippy or slow, this could indicate that your boat has taken on water. In conditions that are calm, open a storage hatch and check it out. *Do not open your boat in conditions that could tip you over, or if waves could wash over the deck.* If there is sufficient bilge water to bail, then do so promptly. If you wait too long and more

water leaks in, then the kayak may sink too low for
bailing.

When a kayak is swamped by large
amounts of bilge water, bailing will not be possible.
Even opening a hatch to check the bilge will only
let more water in. An assisted rescue will be
necessary.

ASSISTED RESCUES:

Kayak over kayak
You will need a second kayak to perform
the "kayak over kayak rescue". The second kayak
should be floating high and largely free of bilge

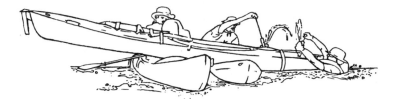

water. An additional rescue kayak is very useful to
provide extra floatation and stability.

Position the rescue boat(s) so the bow of
the swamped boat touches the cockpit of the
rescue boat, making a T. The rescue paddler
should have a firm grip on the swamped boat's
handle. The swamped paddler, swimming, will
position themselves at the intersection of the two
kayaks. The paddlers together will push and pull
the swamped kayak across the rescue kayak(s),
until it is on top and upside down. A hatch or a

drain plug can be opened during this process to let out the water. When the water is drained, then roll the kayak over and push it back in the water. Or the kayak can remain upright while bilge pump(s) are used to remove the water. The swimmer should then reenter their boat and check the bilge for residual water and secure any hatches and drain plugs. Floatation bags in the stern and bow can greatly reduce the effort required to empty a flooded kayak.

Towing

Towing is another important rescue method. A kayak can get loose from its paddler, or a paddler can become sick or weak.

A towrope is an essential piece of rescue equipment. It can be from six feet to twenty-five feet long, with snaps at each end to eliminate the need to tie knots, and an optional elastic section for shock absorption. This feature is handy for long distance towing.

Some towing kits are belt worn, or attached to your life vest with a "quick release" device.

To tow a kayak, your towline needs to be attached to your rear handle. This can be done in advance, or at the time needed by straddling the back deck or swimming to the back deck. The other end of the line attaches to the bow of the kayak that needs to be towed.

Towing is hard work. Be prepared for a workout. If there is a paddler in the other boat, he or she can help by paddling. If that paddler is sick or injured, and not paddling, he or she should be positioned to have a low center of gravity, to in-crease stability. A third kayaker can paddle along side to keep an eye on the sick paddler and assist if there is trouble.

Towing in the surf zone can be difficult and dangerous. Often a kayaker will fall off a boat in the surf zone and need to have it towed to him or her. You must avoid large and breaking waves.

Entanglement can present a serious threat. Having a quick release tow line is wise. A knife should be kept handy, attached to your P.F.D. The rescue of people is always more important than the retrieval of gear.

Towing in moving water like a river or a tidal current can also be dangerous. If you must tow in these conditions use caution and always have a quick release. Do not tow in rapids.

Rescuing a swimmer

Sometimes you must pick up a kayaker who has become a swimmer. This can be a tricky problem for the rescue boater. Carrying a passen-ger on a one-man kayak is a challenge. The swim-mer can capsize your boat if he or she is pan-icked. Putting a person on the stern of your kayak is best, but will make it less stable and slower. Towing a swimmer is harder than towing a boat. There is no easy way to do this, but it must be done sometimes.

14
CHAPTER
SIGNALS

While kayaking, communication can become difficult due to wind noise, crashing surf or great distances. A system of nonverbal signals is practical to use.

You can make these signals easily with your paddle and your hands. A whistle is also good for getting attention; one should be tied to each life vest.

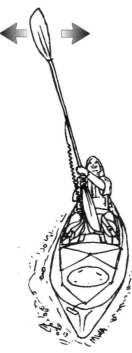

TO SIGNAL FOR HELP...

With your paddle:
Hold it high and wave it over your head back and forth like you are waving a flag.

With your whistle:
You can also use your whistle by blowing three times loudly.

A pattern of three is often used and recognized as a distress signal, Three campfires, three bright colored flags, three horn blasts in groups of three, and *s.o.s... dot dot dot ... dash dash dash ... dot dot dot...* are all common signals for help.

If you see a distress signal, respond promptly and sound the warning to others in your group. Be cautious if helping means you are entering an area of danger. Do not put your self in a position where you will also need to be rescued.

TO SIGNAL A STOP...

Hold the paddle over your head horizontally and pump it up and down as if you are doing pull-ups. Do this if you encounter a danger or an obstacle.

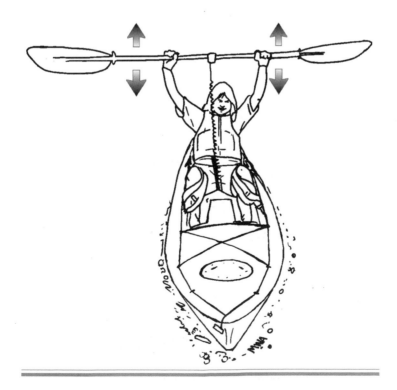

If you see a member of your party ahead of you signaling a stop, then you should signal those behind you.

TO SIGNAL AN ALL CLEAR or GO AHEAD...

Hold the paddle strait up over your head, but do not wave it. In a river or rock garden environment this signal can also mean go straight or center.

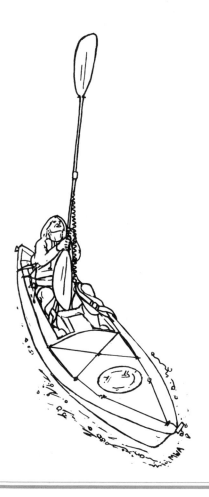

TO SIGNAL A TURN
TO THE RIGHT OR THE LEFT...

Hold the paddle to the left or the right on a high
angle. All these signals can also be used from the
beach to guide incoming paddlers through the surf
zone on a landing.

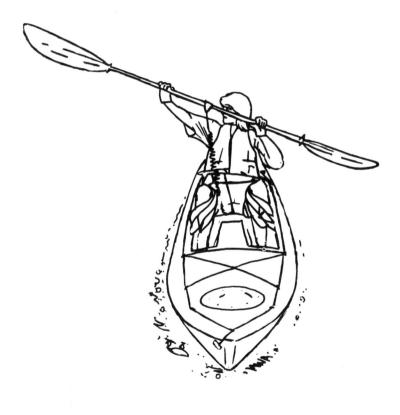

IF YOU NEED TO INDICATE
THAT YOU ARE OK...

or if you need to ask if someone is OK, you can signal by putting a hand on your head making an O. Hold your paddle low because this signal does not use it. You can also signal OK by holding both hands to your head or over your head making a big O.

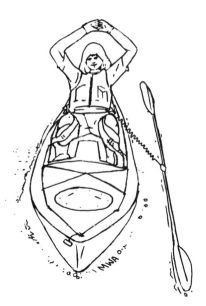

TO GET OTHER PADDLERS ATTENTION...

so that you can signal them, you may need to blow your whistle. Blow it with one blast or more than three blasts to indicate that you just want them to see you. If you are swimming and separated from your paddle, waiving one arm is recognized as a signal of distress for swimmers.

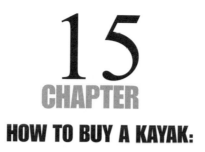

15

CHAPTER

HOW TO BUY A KAYAK:

When purchasing a kayak it is important to ask yourself some questions:

What will I use this kayak for?
Think about your desires and goals. Are you looking for action or adventure, exercise or solitude?

What kind of kayak will meet these goals?

Ask these questions with those who are helping you to make your purchasing decision. A salesperson at kayak shop can be very helpful; but also seek a second opinion from a kayaker friend, an instructor, or consult a magazine or book.
When you have narrowed your choice down to a few models, try them on the water in a safe environment so your focus will be on the test drive. Take your time and make your choice carefully.

Things to consider in a kayak are:
Stability, Speed, Capacity, and
Performance

Generally speaking, a kayak that is...

>*longer will be faster*
>*shorter will be more maneuverable*
>*wider will be more stable.*

Consider your storage needs and compare that to the kayak's storage ability. Visualize yourself using the kayak you are thinking of, like a dress rehearsal.

Choose your accessories with equal care. Try the accessories that you are considering along with the kayaks that you are test paddling.

When you are far from home and in rough condtions you will be depending on your gear. High quality will be necessary.

If you will be using your kayak just once in a while for short distances, then a low quality will be sufficient.

Apply this method to all your accessory purchases. The paddle choice is just as important as the kayak choice. The more you intend to use or depend on the paddle, the higher the quality required.

Also consider how you will transport your kayak. You will need some kind of roof rack. They can be very simple and inexpensive, or very high tech and costly. Make sure that the roof rack is secure, and that the kayak tied to it is also secure. Some roof racks are made only to fit certain cars. Other racks will fit all cars. Make sure that the rack is the right kind for your car, by reading the instructions carefully.

When you have made your purchase it is

time to get started. Go with a club, tour group, or experienced buddies.

Wear your life vest, particularly if you are a beginner or a poor swimmer. The best place to store the life vest is to wear it. If not, have it ready for instant use.

Paddle in conditions where you are comfortable. Do not paddle in conditions that frighten you.

Most of all have fun and enjoy the camaraderie or the solitude. Share your experience and knowledge with others. There is a lot of room for this new branch of the sport to grow, and for you to grow with it.

GLOSSARY

BACKREST: *AN ACCESSORY TO SUPPORT THE BACK*

BILGE PUMP: *A DEVICE FOR SUCKING WATER OUT OF THE BOAT*

BILGE WATER: *THE WATER INSIDE YOUR KAYAK*

BOW: *THE FRONT OF THE BOAT*

BOWLINE: *A GENERAL PURPOSE ROPE ATTACHED TO THE BOW*

BROACH: *SURFING SIDEWAYS ON A WAVE*

BUNGIE NET: *LACE WORK OF SHOCK CORD TO HOLD ITEMS*

CARGO DECK: *A DEPRESSION IN THE DECK, OFTEN WITH STRAPS*

COCKPIT: *THE DEPRESSION IN THE BOAT WHERE YOU SIT*

DECK: *THE TOP OF THE KAYAK*

DECK BAG: *A NET BAG SECURED TO THE DECK FOR STORAGE*

DECK LINE: *ROPE THAT RUNS ALONG THE DECK FOR HANDHOLDS*

DIVE FLAG: *A FLAG TO INDICATE THAT A DIVER IS UNDER WATER*

DRAIN PLUG: *A CORK IN THE DECK TO LET OUT BILGEWATER*

DRY BAG: *A WATERPROOF SACK*

DYE MARKER: *SPREADS ON THE WATER TO MAKE A SIGNAL*

ESKIMO-ROLL: *METHOD USED TO RIGHT AN UPSIDE DOWN KAYAK*

FEATHERED: *PADDLE BLADES AT ANGLES OF UP TO 90 DEGREES*

FERRY: *TO CUT DIAGONALLY ACROSS A STRONG CURRENT*

FLARE: *PYROTECHNIC DEVICE TO CREATE AN ILLUMINOUS SIGNAL*

FLOAT BAGS: *AIR BAGS TO KEEP A SWAMPED KAYAK AFLOAT*

FLOAT PLAN: *A DETAILED PLAN OF YOUR TRIP*

FOOTWELLS: *THE PLACE FOR FEET*

GUNWHALE: *THE OUTER EDGE OF THE COCKPIT*

HANDLES: *TOGGLES ON THE BOW AND STERN*

HATCH: *AN ACCESS PORT INTO THE INTERIOR OF THE KAYAK*

HULL: *THE BOTTOM OF THE KAYAK*

KAYAK: *A PADDLE CRAFT FOR ONE OR TWO PEOPLE*

KNEE STRAPS: *ACCESSORY FOR THE LEGS TO GRIP THE KAYAK*

LEG LEASH: *A CORD THAT ATTACHES A KAYAK TO THE PADDLER*

LIFE JACKET: *A FLOTATION DEVICE WORN FOR SAFETY*

LIFELINE: *A ROPE THAT ATTACHES THE PADDLER TO THE KAYAK*

MOOR: *TO ANCHOR YOUR KAYAK*

PADDLE: *A DOUBLE BLADED PROPULSION DEVICE*

PADDLE LEASH: *A CORD TO ATTACH THE PADDLE TO THE KAYAK*

PFD: *PERSONAL FLOATATION DEVICE, LIFE VEST*

PORTAGE: *TO CARRY YOUR KAYAK OVERLAND*

PUT IN: *THE PLACE WHERE A PADDLING TRIP STARTS*

RACK STRAPS: *TIE DOWNS TO SECURE YOUR KAYAK*

ROCK GARDEN: *A SURF ZONE AREA WITH LOTS OF ROCKS*

ROD HOLDER: *A DEVICE MOUNTED TO THE DECK TO HOLD A POLE*

ROOF RACK: *TWO BARS ON TOP OF A CAR TO TIE KAYAKS TO*

RUDDER: *A FOOT CONTROLLED DEVICE FOR STEERING*

SCUPPER: *A HOLE IN THE DECK THAT DRAINS INTO THE SEA*

SEA ANCHOR: *A PARACHUTE FOR THE WATER TO PREVENT DRIFT*

SEE RESCUE: *SIGNAL THAT CAN BE SEEN FROM ABOVE*

SIGNAL MIRROR: *A MIRROR FOR FLASHING A DISTRESS SIGNAL*

SKEG: *A FIN ON THE BOTTOM OF THE BOAT*

SMOKE MARKER: *PYROTECHNIC TO CREATE A SMOKE SIGNAL*

SOFT RACK: *PADS TO PUT ON YOUR CAR ROOF FOR YOUR KAYAK*

STERN: *THE BACK OF THE BOAT*

STING AIDE: *REDUCES PAIN OF STINGS FROM MARINE ORGANISMS*

STRAP EYE: *AN OPEN RING ON THE DECK FOR ATTACHMENTS*

TAKE OUT: *THE PLACE WHERE A PADDLING TRIP ENDS*

TANKWELL: *A RECESSED STORAGE AREA ON DECK FOR CARGO*

TIDE CHART: *SHOWS THE TIDES OF EACH DAY FOR THAT REGION*

INDEX

A

ACCESSORIES: CHAPTER 3, 12, 82

ANCHOR: 52-54

B

BACKREST: 8, 14

BACKWARDS, PADDLING: 27, 29, 30

BAILING: (see BILGE WATER)

BILGE PUMPS: 66, 71

BILGE WATER: 8, 71

BODY POSTURE: 34-35, 56

BOWLINE: 13

BRACING: 34-35, 46

BROACHING: (see SIDEWAYS)

BUNGIE NET/CORD: 12, 14

C

CAMPING: 9, 58-59

CAPSIZING: 5, 16, 23-24, 34, 45-46, 52, 56-57, 74

CHECKLISTS: 18-20, 60-61, 66

CLOTHING: 19

COCKPIT: 7, 24

CURRENT: 41, 43, 63

D

DECK LINES: 14

DIVE FLAG: 53

DIVING: 53-54

DOCKING: 13, 36-37

DRAIN PLUG: 13, 21, 73

DYE MARKER: 66

E

ESKIMO-ROLL: 5

F

FEATHERED PADDLE: 28, 29

FERRY: 41

FINS: 9

FISHING: 9, 51-52

FLOAT BAGS: 66 (GLOSSARY)

FLOAT PLAN: 67-69 CHAPTER 11

FOOTWELLS: 23, 25

G

GROUP PADDLING: 64, 67-69, CHAPTER 14

GUNWHALE: 12 (GLOSSARY)

MANUFACTURERS OF
SIT-ON-TOP KAYAKS

FROM THE GROWING LIST OF SIT-ON-TOP MANUFACTURERS. CHECK OUT THEIR WEB SITE OR CALL & REQUEST A CATALOG

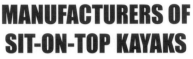
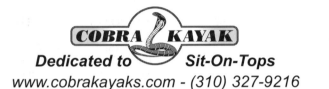
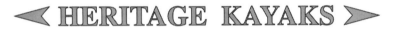
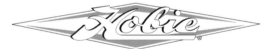
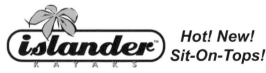

WHERE TO GET A SIT-ON-TOP KAYAK

FROM THE GROWING LIST OF SIT-ON-TOP DEALERS AND OUTFITTERS NEAR YOU:

ALABAMA

ALABAMA OUTDOORS
3054 INDEPENDENCE DR
BIRMINGHAM, AL 35209
(205) 870-1919

ALASKA

SUSITNA EXPEDITIONS
PO BOX 520243
SUNRISE DRIVE
BIG LAKE, AK 99652
1(800) 891-6916
fax: (907) 892-7727
kayaker@mtaonline.net

ARIZONA

DESERT RIVER OUTFITTER
2649 HWY 95 STE 23
BULLHEAD CITY, AZ 86440
(520) 763-3033
(888) KAYAK-33

TWIN FINN INC
BOX 4780
811 VISTA AVE
PAGE, AZ 86040
(520) 645-3114
twinfinn@page-lakepowell.com

ARKANSAS

ADAM'S OUFITTER
113 W. WALNUT ST
ROGERS, AR 72756
(501) 636-1024

CALIFORNIA

SAILBOATS OF BAKERSFIELD
3100 UNION AVE
BAKERSFIELD, CA 93305
(661) 322-9178 fax: (661) 322-3411
sailboatbak@lightspeed.net

CARLSBAD PADDLE SPORTS
2780 CARLSBAD BLVD
CARLSBAD, CA 92008
(760) 434-8686
kayak@inetaccess.com
www.carslbadpaddle.com

ADVENTURE SPORTS
6040 FAIR OAKS BLVD
CARMICHAEL, CA 95608
(916) 971-1800

ACTION WATERSPORTS
4144 LINCOLN BLVD
MARINA DEL REY, CA 90291
(310) 827-2233 fax: (310) 305-8046
www.actionwatersports.com

PADDLE POWER
1500 W BALBOA BLVD
NEW PORT BEACH, CA 92663
(949) 675-1215
fax:(949) 675-7131

PADDLE SPORTS
100 STATE ST
SANTA BARBARA, CA 93101
(805) 899-4925 fax: (805) 568-0583

WIND TOYS
3019 SANTA ROSA AVE
SANTA ROSA, CA 95407
(707) 542-7245
(800) 499-SAIL

CALIFORNIA (CON'T)

CENTRAL COAST KAYAKS
1879 SHELL BEACH ROAD
SHELL BEACH, CA 93449
(805) 773-3500
fax: (805) 773-9767

OFF THE BEACH BOATS
15 CALLE DEL MAR #3
STINSON BEACH, CA 94970
(415) 868-9445
fax (415) 868-9798

COLORADO

ALPEN GLOW
885 LUPINE ST #B
GOLDEN, CO 80401
(303) 277-0133
fax: (303) 277-0138

CONNECTICUT

SKI MARKET
432 BUCKLAND HILLS DR
MANCHESTER, CT 06040
(860) 644-6200 fax: (860) 644-7697

THE SMALL BOAT SHOP
144 WATER ST
NORWALK, CT 06854
(203) 854-5223
www.thesmallboatshop.com

DELAWARE

EAST OF MAUI
104 ST LOUIS ST
DEWEY BEACH, DE 19971
(302) 227-4703 fax: (302) 227-4708
eastofmaui@erols.com
www.eastofmaui.com

FLORIDA

ACTION WATERSPORTS
402 PROGRESS RD
AUBURNDALE, FL 33823
(941) 967-4148
fax: (941) 967-0070
dsims1@gte.net

FLORIDA (CON'T)

WATERPLAY
2550 S BAYSHORE DR
COCONUT GROVE, FL 33133
(305) 860-0888 fax: (305) 860-1199
sales@water-play.com

CANOE OUTFITTERS OF FLORIDA
8900 WEST INDIANTOWN RD
JUPITER, FL 33478
(561) 746-7053 fax: (561) 744-5169
(888) 272-1257 cancof@aol.com
www.canoes-kayaks-florida.com

JUPITER OUTDOOR CENTER
18091 NORTH A1A
JUPITER, FL 33477
(561) 747-9666
rick@jupiteroutdoorcenter.com

AQUA EAST SURF SHOP
696 ATLANTIC BLVD
NEPTUNE BEACH, FL 32266
(904) 246-2550

ADVENTURE TIMES KAYAKS
521 NORTHLAKE BLVD
NORTH PALM BEACH, FL 33408
(561) 881-7218
1-888-KAYAK-FL
fax: (561) 844-1164
kayakfla@aol.com

COASTAL KAYAKS
4255 A1A South
ST AUGUSTINE, FL 32084
(904) 471-4144
www.coastalkayaks.com
cokayaks@aol.com

CANOE COUNTRY OUTFITTERS
6493 54 AVE North
ST PETERSBURG, FL 33709
(727) 545-4554
fax: (727) 545-4554

SILENT SPORTS OUTFITTERS
2301 TAMIAMI TRAIL NORTH
NOKOMIS, FL 34275
(941) 966-5477
fax: (941) 966-0928

GEORGIA

GO WITH THE FLOW SPORTS INC
4 ELIZABETH WAY
ROSWELL, GA 30075
(770) 992-3200 fax: (770) 992-9033

HAWAIIAN ISLANDS - OAHU

GO BANANAS
799 KAPAHULU AVE
HONOLULU, HI 96816
(808) 737-9514

TWOGOOD KAYAKS HAWAII, INC
345 HAHANI ST
KAILUA, HI 96734
(808) 262-5656 fax:(808)261-3111
twogood@aloha.com

KAILUA SAILBOARDS
& KAYAKS INC.
130 KAILUA RD
KAILUA, HI 96734
(808) 262-2555 fax: (808) 261-7341
watersports@aloha.net

HAWAIIAN ISLANDS - MAUI

SOUTH PACIFIC KAYAKS
2439 South KIHEI RD #101 B
KIHEI, MAUI, HI 96753
(808) 875-4848 fax: (808) 875-4691
seakayak@maui.net
www.mauikayak.com

MAUI SEA KAYAKING
P.O. BOX 106
PU'UNENE, HI 96784
(808) 572-6299 / kayaking@maui.net
www.maui.net/~kayaking

HAWAIIAN ISLANDS - KAUA'I

KAYAK KAUA'I OUTBOUND
HIKE-BIKE-CAMP-PADDLE
TOURS AND RENTALS
KAPA'A (808) 822-9179
HANALEI (808) 826-9844
toll free: (800) 437-3507
info@kayakkauai.com
www.kayakkauai.com

HAWAIIAN ISLANDS - KAUA'I

OUTFITTERS KAUAI
2827 A POIPU RD
KOLOA, KAUAI, HI 96756
(808) 742-9667OR (888) 742-9887
info@outfitterskauai.com
www.outfitterskauai.com

INDIANA

OUTPOST SPORTS
3602 N GRAPE RD
MISHAWAKA, IN 46545
(219) 259-1000

IOWA

BOULEVARD SPORTS
4211 CHAMBERLAIN DR
DES MOINES, IA 50312
(515) 255-8433 fax: (515) 255-3879

MAINE

KITTERY TRADING POST
301 US RTE1
KITTERY, ME 03904-0904
(207) 439-2700 fax: (207) 439-8001

MARYLAND

SUNNY'S OUTDOOR STORE, INC
2157-B YORK RD
TIMONIUM, MD 21093
(410) 561-7885

EAST OF MAUI
2303 FOREST DRIVE
SUITE E
ANNAPOLIS, MD 21401
(410) 573-9463 fax: (410) 573-9465
eastofmaui@erols.com
www.eastofmaui.com

MASSACHUSETTS

SKI MARKET - BOSTON
860 COMMONWEALTH AVE
BOSTON, MA 02215
(617) 731-6100
fax: (617) 232-4004

MASSACHUSETTS (CON'T)

SKI MARKET - BRAINTREE
400 FRANKLIN ST
BRAINTREE, MA 02184
(781) 848-3733
fax: (781) 848-7499

YANKEE AQUATICS
17 SCHOOL STREET
EASTHAMPTON, MA 01027
(413) 527-5237

**CHARLES RIVER
CANOE & KAYAK**
2401 COMMONWEALTH AVE
NEWTON, MA 02466
(617) 965-5110
info@ski-paddle.com
www.ski-paddle.com

SALTMARSH SEAKAYAK
589 FISHER ROAD
N DARTMOUTH, MA 02747
(508) 636-3007
fax: (508) 636-3007
hiyi1939@aol.com

SKI MARKET - PEMBROKE
CHRISTMAS TREE SHOPS
RT #139
PEMBROKE, MA 02359
(781) 826-1155
fax: (781) 826-6330

MICHIGAN

LUMBERTOWN CANOE & KAYAK
276 OTTAWA STREET
MUSKEGON, MI 49442
(616) 728-2276

MINNESOTA

MINNESOTA SCHOOL OF DIVING
712 WASHINGTON ST
BRAINERD, MN 56401
(218) 829-5953
fax: (218) 828-7909
1(800) OK-SCUBA
www.mndiving.com

MONTANA

BIKOLOGY & CANOE WORLD
155 N MAIN STREET
KALISPELL, MT 59901
(406) 755-6755
fax: (406) 755-6755

NEVADA

P & S HARDWARE
905 WEST FIFTH STREET
RENO, NV 89503
(702) 329-1392
fax: (702) 329-1392

NEW HAMPSHIRE

SKI MARKET - MANCHESTER
717 SOUTH WILLOW STREET
MANCHESTER, NH 03103
(603) 647-1212 fax: (603) 622-3888

WINNIPESAUKEE KAYAK
17 BAY STREET
WOLFBORO, NH 03894
(603) 569-9926 fax: (603) 569-0200

NEW JERSEY

JERSEY PADDLER
1756 ROUTE 88
BRICK, NJ 08724
1(888) 22-KAYAK

TI KAYAKS
5006 LANDIS AVE
SEA ISLE CITY, NJ 08243
(609) 263-0805

ISLAND KAYAK COMPANY
1116 STONE HARBOR BLVD
STONE HARBOR, NJ 08247
(609) 368-1001 fax: (609) 368-5318
kayaknj@algorithms.com

ISLAND SURF & SAIL
3304 LONGBEACH BLVD
BRANT BEACH, NJ 08008
(609) 494-5553 fax: (609) 494-5150
Tdeakyne@msn.com
www.Islandsurf-sail.com

NEW MEXICO

OUTBACK GEAR
100 WASHINGTON
CIMARRON, NM 87714
(505) 376-2121 (888) 311CAMP
www.outbackgear.com

NEW YORK

CANANDAIGUA SAILBOARDING
11 LAKESHORE DR
CANANDAIGUA, NY 14424
(716) 394-8150

EMPIRE KAYAKS
4 EMPIRE BLVD
ISLAND PARK, NY 11558
(516) 889-8300 fax: (516) 897-9366

PECONIC PADDLER
89 PECONIC AVE
RIVERHEAD, NY 11901
(516) 727-9895

OAK ORCHARD
CANOE & KAYAK EXPERTS
40 STATE ST
PITTSFORD, NY 14534
(716) 586-5990
OR: 2133 EAGLE HARBOR RD
WATERPORT, NY 14571
(716) 682-4849

MAIN BEACH SURF & SAIL
MONTAUK HWY
WAINSCOTT, NY 11975
(516) 537-2716 fax: (516) 537-6310

SKI MARKET - WILLIAMSVILLE
TRANSITOWN PLAZA
WILLIAMSVILLE, NY 14221
(716) 634-8160
fax: (716) 634-4566

NORTH CAROLINA

KITTY HAWK SPORTS
3933 SOUTH CROATAN
NAGS HEAD, NC 27959
(252) 441-6800 fax: (252) 441-5117

NORTH CAROLINA (CON'T)

HERRINGS OUTDOOR SPORTS
PO BOX 2098
SURF CITY, NC 28445
(910) 328-3291

CAPE FEAR OUTFITTERS
1934 A EASTWOOD RD
WILMINGTON, NC 28403
(910) 256-1258 fax: (910) 256-1259

OHIO

OUTBACK GEAR
408 EASTWOOD MALL
NILES, OH 44446
1 (888) 311-CAMP
www.outbackgear.com

OREGON

CENTRAL COAST
WATERSPORTS
PO BOX 435
FLORENCE, OR 97439
(541) 997-1812

PENNSYLVANIA

OUTBACK GEAR
JOHNSTOWN GALLERIA
JOHNSTOWN, PA 15904
(814) 262-6115 / (888) 311CAMP
www.outbackgear.com

RHODE ISLAND

OCEANS & PONDS
217 OCEAN AVE
BLOCK ISLAND, RI 02807
(401) 466-5131 fax: (401) 466-2137
1morecast@ids.net

THE KAYAK CENTRE
9 PHILLIPS STREET
WICKFORD, RI 02852
(401) 295-4400
1(888) SEA-KAYAK
www.kayakcentre.com
funn@kayakcenter.com

SOUTH CAROLINA

OUTSIDE HILTON HEAD
THE PLAZA AT SHELTER COVE
BOX H
HILTON HEAD ISLAND, SC 29928
(843) 686-6996 (800) 686-6996
fax: (843) 686-6006
www.outsidehiltonhead.com

TEXAS

**AUSTIN OUTDOOR
GEAR & GUIDANCE
WILDERNESS SUPPLY**
3411 NORTH INTRSTATE HWY 35
AUSTIN, TX 78722
(512) 473-2644
fax: (512) 473-2628
aogg2@gte.net

COASTAL PADDLER
4099 B CALDER
BEAUMONT, TX 77706
(409) 899-4397 fax: (409) 896-5404
coastalpad@aol.com

WILDERNESS FUNISHINGS INC.
5420 MANOR DR
SUGARLAND, TX 77479
(281) 403-9013
www.wildfur.com

VERMONT

SMALL BOAT EXCHANGE
16 KILBURN ST
BURLINGTON, VT 05401
(802) 864-5437 fax: (802) 658-8057

VIRGINIA

WILD RIVER OUTFITTERS
3636 VIRGINIA BEACH BLVD #108
VIRGINIA BEACH, VA 23452
(757) 431-8566 fax: (757) 340-1098
mail@wildriveroutfitters.com
www.wildriveroutfitters.com

WASHINGTON

KAYAK ACADEMY
2512 NE 95TH STREET
SEATTLE, WA 98115
(206) 527-1825
kayak@halcyon.com
www.halcyon.com/kayak/

WISCONSIN

COONTAIL WATERSPORTS
5466 PARK ST
BOULDER JUNCTION, WI 54512
(715) 385-O250 fax: (715) 385-2731
www.coontailsports.com

If you would like to list your kayak club, school, store, dealership, or manufacturing business in a future edition of
SIT-ON-TOP KAYAKING, A BEGINNER'S GUIDE
or if you are unable to locate additional copies of
SIT-ON-TOP KAYAKING, A BEGINNER'S GUIDE
contact the publisher at
**GeoOdyssey Publications
P.O. Box 25441
Rochester, NY 14625
Toll free: (877) 893-1726
email: geodysy@aol.com**

LEARN MORE ABOUT SIT-ON-TOP KAYAKING AND SHARE YOUR OWN KAYAKING ADVENTURES WHEN YOU CHECK OUT OUR WEB SITE AT:

www.Sit-on-topKayaking.com